CONTENTS

MIND SCRATCH 500+ AMAZING WORKOUT FACTS

Well, you have got this far so keep reading to find all the inspiration you could ever need to take that step into the world of the workout. Dip into those curiosities about all of the most popular exercises, find the ones that suit you and put yourself together a workout routine to fit your lifestyle.

In this delightful book are over 500 facts about exercises to train every part of your body, top to toe.

The book is written in no particular order, so you can read it any way you choose, read front to back, in reverse or jump around any way you please. It makes a great companion piece to take on a long journey, have a read through with a friend, give yourself that extra push to workout in the gym (or at home), or have a flick through to help your tired eyes catch some zzz's.

There are almost limitless ways to enjoy this fascinating book of exercise facts, so take that first, small step on your fitness journey and indulge your curiosity.

PUSH UP

- Push-ups are a fundamental bodyweight exercise that primarily targets the muscles of the chest, shoulders, and triceps.

- The push-up is a compound exercise, engaging multiple muscle groups simultaneously, including the core and lower body to a lesser extent.

- Variations of push-ups include standard push-ups, wide grip, narrow grip, decline, and incline push-ups, allowing for targeting different muscle groups.

- Proper form is crucial for push-ups to prevent strain on the shoulders and lower back. The body should form a straight line from head to heels.

- Push-ups are an excellent bodyweight exercise for building upper body strength and endurance.

- They can be modified for different fitness levels by adjusting the incline or performing them on the knees.

- Push-ups are often used as a benchmark exercise to assess upper body strength and overall fitness.

- Adding variations like explosive or plyometric push-ups can increase the intensity and provide cardiovascular benefits.

- Push-ups contribute to improved shoulder stability and mobility.

- This exercise helps develop scapular retraction and protraction, essential for overall shoulder health.

- Push-ups engage the serratus anterior, a muscle important for shoulder blade movement and stability.

- Performing push-ups regularly can help improve posture by strengthening the muscles that support the spine.

- Push-ups can be done virtually anywhere, requiring no special equipment, making them a convenient and accessible exercise.

LUNGE

- Lunges are a versatile lower body exercise that targets the muscles in the legs, including the quadriceps, hamstrings, and glutes.

- There are several variations of lunges, including forward lunges, reverse lunges, walking lunges, and side lunges.

- Lunges also engage the core muscles, helping to improve overall stability and balance.

- One of the primary benefits of lunges is their ability to strengthen and tone the muscles around the hips, thighs, and buttocks.

- Lunges are a functional exercise that mimics many everyday movements, making them beneficial for improving overall athleticism.

- Proper form is crucial when performing lunges to avoid strain on the knees and ensure maximum effectiveness.

- Lunges can be performed with body weight only, or they can be enhanced by holding weights such as dumbbells or a barbell.

- Including lunges in your workout routine can help improve flexibility and range of motion in the hips and knees.

- The dynamic nature of lunges makes them effective for warming up before more intense workouts.

- Lunges are a unilateral exercise, meaning they work one leg at a time, helping to address muscle imbalances.

- Incorporating lunges into your fitness routine can contribute to better posture by strengthening the muscles responsible for maintaining an upright position.

- Adding variations like jumping lunges can increase the intensity of the exercise, providing cardiovascular benefits and enhancing overall agility.

BURPEE

- The burpee is a full-body exercise that combines elements of strength training and cardiovascular conditioning.

- A basic burpee involves a sequence of movements, including a squat, plank, push-up, squat thrust, and a jump.

- Burpees are an efficient and effective exercise for burning calories due to their high intensity and incorporation of multiple muscle groups.

- This exercise engages muscles in the legs, core, chest, shoulders, and arms.

- Burpees are often used in High-Intensity Interval Training (HIIT) workouts for their ability to elevate heart rate rapidly.

- Variations of burpees exist, allowing for modifications based on fitness levels and goals, such as adding a jump at the end or incorporating dumbbells.

- Burpees are a great functional exercise, as they mimic movements often used in everyday activities.

- Performing burpees regularly can contribute to increased muscular endurance and cardiovascular fitness.

- The explosive nature of the jump in a burpee helps enhance power and explosiveness.

- Burpees can be adapted for individuals with joint issues or beginners by reducing the impact or eliminating certain components of the exercise.

- Including burpees in a workout routine can lead to improved agility and coordination.

- Burpees require no special equipment, making them a convenient bodyweight exercise that can be done anywhere.

- This exercise is time-efficient, providing a quick and intense workout option for those with busy schedules.

DIP

- Dips are a bodyweight exercise that primarily targets the muscles of the upper body, including the chest, shoulders, and triceps.

- There are two main types of dips: parallel bar dips and bench dips. Parallel bar dips involve using parallel bars, while bench dips are performed using a bench or sturdy surface.

- Parallel bar dips engage the chest and shoulders more intensely, while bench dips place greater emphasis on the triceps.

- Dips are considered a compound exercise, involving multiple joints and muscle groups in the movement.

- Proper form is essential for dips to avoid unnecessary strain on the shoulders and to maximize effectiveness. The body should be kept upright, and elbows should be at a 90-degree angle.

- Dips are an excellent exercise for developing upper body strength and muscular endurance.

- This exercise also engages the muscles of the core, as the body must stabilize during the movement.

- Dips can be adapted for different fitness levels by adjusting the difficulty level or using assistance from a dip machine or resistance bands.

- Variations of dips include adding weight with a dipping belt or using different hand positions to target various muscle groups.

- Dips contribute to improved shoulder stability and flexibility.

- Including dips in a workout routine can help build a well-rounded and balanced upper body.

- Dips are often used in calisthenics and bodyweight training programs due to their effectiveness and simplicity.

BODYWEIGHT ROW

- Bodyweight rows, also known as inverted rows or Australian pull-ups, are a strength training exercise targeting the muscles of the upper back, including the latissimus dorsi and rhomboids.

- This exercise can be performed using a horizontal bar, Smith machine, suspension trainer, or even a sturdy table at home.

- Bodyweight rows are a compound exercise, engaging multiple muscles in the upper body, including the biceps, rear deltoids, and traps.

- Proper form is crucial for bodyweight rows to ensure effective muscle engagement and prevent strain on the lower back. The body should form a straight line from head to heels.

- Adjusting the angle of the body or the height of the bar allows for modification of difficulty, making bodyweight rows suitable for various fitness levels.

- This exercise helps improve posture by strengthening the muscles responsible for scapular retraction.

- Bodyweight rows are an effective alternative to traditional pull-ups, allowing individuals to build upper body strength without the need for a vertical pulling motion.

- Including bodyweight rows in a workout routine contributes to enhanced grip strength, as the exercise requires holding onto a bar or handles.

- The inverted position of bodyweight rows promotes blood flow to the upper body and can be beneficial for shoulder health.

- Variations, such as one-arm bodyweight rows or incorporating pauses at the top of the movement, can add complexity and increase the intensity of the exercise.

- Bodyweight rows are a functional exercise that mimics pulling movements used in daily activities, making them valuable for overall fitness.

BAR HANG

- Bar hangs, also known as passive hangs or dead hangs, involve gripping a horizontal bar and letting your body hang freely.

- This simple yet effective exercise primarily targets the muscles in the upper body, including the forearms, grip, shoulders, and upper back.

- Bar hangs can be performed on various types of bars, such as pull-up bars, monkey bars, or gymnastic rings.

- The exercise helps improve grip strength, which is beneficial for various activities in daily life and other exercises.

- Bar hangs decompress the spine and stretch the shoulders, providing relief for individuals with tightness or discomfort in the upper body.

- Performing bar hangs can contribute to better shoulder mobility and flexibility by allowing the shoulder joints to move through a full range of motion.

- Hanging from a bar engages the muscles of the core as they work to stabilize the body in the hanging position.

- Bar hangs are beginner-friendly and suitable for individuals of different fitness levels. They can be easily modified by adjusting the duration of the hang or using assistance if needed.

- Hanging from a bar elongates the spine, promoting good posture and counteracting the effects of sitting for extended periods.

- Incorporating bar hangs into a workout routine can help activate the muscles around the shoulder blades, improving scapular mobility and stability.

- Bar hangs are a low-impact exercise, making them suitable for individuals with joint issues or those looking for a recovery activity.

- Holding a bar hang challenges the muscles in the hands and fingers, contributing to improved dexterity and hand strength.

PULL UP

- Pull-ups are a classic and effective upper body exercise that targets the muscles of the back, particularly the latissimus dorsi.

- The primary muscles engaged in pull-ups include the latissimus dorsi, rhomboids, rear deltoids, biceps, and forearms.

- Pull-ups are a compound exercise, involving movement at multiple joints, making them highly efficient for building upper body strength.

- Proper form is crucial for pull-ups to maximize effectiveness and prevent injury. This includes a full range of motion, starting from a dead hang and pulling until the chin is above the bar.

- Pull-ups can be performed with various grip positions, such as wide grip, close grip, or neutral grip, targeting different muscle groups.

- This exercise contributes to improved grip strength, as the hands and forearms play a significant role in maintaining a secure grip on the bar.

- Pull-ups are an excellent measure of relative upper body strength, as they require lifting your entire body weight.

- Beginners can use assisted pull-up machines or resistance bands to gradually build strength and work towards unassisted pull-ups.

- Pull-ups are a versatile exercise that can be performed on various types of bars, including pull-up bars, gymnastic rings, or even tree branches.

- Including pull-ups in your workout routine helps develop a V-shaped torso by targeting the muscles of the upper back and shoulders.

- The exercise activates the core muscles, contributing to overall core strength and stability.

- Pull-ups can be part of a calisthenics training program, providing a challenging bodyweight exercise without the need for additional equipment.

CHIN UP

- Chin-ups are a type of pull-up exercise that targets the muscles of the upper back, particularly the latissimus dorsi, and also heavily engages the biceps.

- The primary difference between pull-ups and chin-ups is the grip. In chin-ups, the palms face towards the body (underhand grip), while pull-ups typically have an overhand grip.

- Chin-ups involve the activation of the biceps more than pull-ups due to the supinated (palms facing towards the body) grip.

- Proper form is essential for chin-ups to ensure maximum muscle engagement and to avoid unnecessary strain on the shoulders and wrists.

- Chin-ups are a compound exercise, recruiting multiple muscle groups such as the rhomboids, rear deltoids, and various forearm muscles.

- Like pull-ups, chin-ups are an excellent measure of upper body strength as they require lifting your entire body weight.

- Beginners can use assistance from bands or machines to gradually build strength and work towards unassisted chin-ups.

- Chin-ups contribute to improved grip strength, as the exercise challenges the muscles in the hands and forearms.

- Chin-ups can be performed on various types of bars, providing versatility in training environments.

- Including chin-ups in your workout routine helps develop a well-rounded and sculpted upper body, emphasizing the biceps and upper back.

- Chin-ups activate the core muscles, promoting overall core strength and stability.

- Incorporating different variations of chin-ups, such as weighted chin-ups or eccentric chin-ups, can add complexity and intensity to the exercise.

PLANK

- The plank is a static core exercise that involves maintaining a straight line from head to heels while supporting the body on the forearms and toes.

- Planks primarily target the muscles of the core, including the rectus abdominis, transverse abdominis, obliques, and the muscles of the lower back.

- Proper form is crucial for planks to effectively engage the core and prevent strain on the lower back. The body should be in a straight line, and the core muscles should be actively contracted.

- Planks can be modified to suit various fitness levels, with options such as forearm planks, high planks, side planks, and plank variations with leg or arm lifts.

- The exercise is isometric, meaning it involves holding a static position, which helps improve muscular endurance in the core.

- Planks engage not only the core but also the muscles in the shoulders, arms, and legs, making them a full-body workout.

- Planks are beneficial for improving posture by strengthening the muscles that support the spine.

- Including planks in a workout routine can contribute to increased stability and balance, as the exercise requires maintaining a stable position.

- Planks are often used in rehabilitation programs for individuals recovering from lower back issues, as they promote core strength without putting excessive stress on the spine.

- Planks are time-efficient, providing a quick and effective workout for the core muscles without the need for additional equipment.

- This exercise helps to strengthen the muscles around the pelvis, which is beneficial for overall pelvic stability.

HIP BRIDGE HOLD

- The hip bridge hold is a static exercise that involves lifting the hips toward the ceiling while maintaining a straight line from the shoulders to the knees.

- This exercise primarily targets the muscles of the glutes, including the gluteus maximus, as well as the hamstrings and lower back.

- Proper form is essential for hip bridge holds to engage the targeted muscles and prevent unnecessary strain on the lower back. The body should form a straight line, and the core muscles should be activated.

- Hip bridge holds are effective for activating and strengthening the posterior chain, which includes the muscles on the backside of the body.

- The exercise can be modified by performing single-leg hip bridge holds or by adding resistance such as a barbell or resistance band for increased intensity.

- Hip bridge holds contribute to improved hip mobility and flexibility.

- Including this exercise in a workout routine can help address muscle imbalances in the hips and pelvis.

- Hip bridge holds are often used in rehabilitation programs for individuals recovering from lower back or hip issues, as they provide a low-impact way to strengthen the posterior chain.

- The exercise engages the core muscles, promoting overall core strength and stability.

- Hip bridge holds can be included in warm-up routines to activate the glutes and prepare the body for more intense exercises.

- Performing hip bridge holds regularly can contribute to better posture by strengthening the muscles that support the spine.

- This exercise is suitable for individuals of various fitness levels and can be adapted to meet specific needs, making it a versatile addition to workout programs.

HANGING KNEE TUCK

- Hanging knee tucks are a dynamic core exercise that involves hanging from a bar and bringing the knees toward the chest.

- This exercise primarily targets the abdominal muscles, including the rectus abdominis and the lower part of the obliques.

- Proper form is essential for hanging knee tucks to effectively engage the core and prevent unnecessary strain on the shoulders. Maintain control throughout the movement.

- Hanging knee tucks can be performed on various types of bars, such as pull-up bars or gymnastic rings.

- The exercise can be modified to suit different fitness levels by adjusting the difficulty level or incorporating variations, such as hanging knee raises or straight leg raises.

- Hanging knee tucks help improve hip flexor flexibility as the knees are brought toward the chest.

- This exercise also engages the muscles of the upper body, including the shoulders, forearms, and grip strength.

- Hanging knee tucks are an effective way to target the lower abdominal region, which can be challenging to engage with traditional abdominal exercises.

- Including hanging knee tucks in a workout routine can contribute to increased core strength and stability.

- This exercise requires coordination and balance, promoting overall body awareness.

- Hanging knee tucks can be part of a comprehensive core training program, helping to develop a well-rounded and sculpted midsection.

- Beginners can start with bent knee variations and gradually progress to straight leg variations as they build strength.

HOLLOW BODY ROCKING

- Hollow body rocking is a dynamic core exercise that involves creating a "hollow" shape with the body and rocking back and forth.

- This exercise targets the entire core, including the rectus abdominis, transverse abdominis, and obliques.

- Proper form is crucial for hollow body rocking to effectively engage the core and prevent strain on the lower back. The lower back should be pressed into the floor, and the legs and upper body should be lifted slightly.

- Hollow body rocking helps improve core strength and stability by challenging the muscles to maintain the hollow position while in motion.

- The exercise also engages the hip flexors, contributing to improved flexibility in the hips.

- Hollow body rocking can be adapted to different fitness levels by adjusting the difficulty level or incorporating variations, such as rocking from side to side.

- This exercise promotes body awareness, as individuals need to concentrate on maintaining a specific body position throughout the movement.

- Hollow body rocking is a low-impact exercise, making it suitable for individuals with lower back issues or those looking for an alternative to high-impact core exercises.

- Including hollow body rocking in a workout routine can contribute to better posture by strengthening the muscles that support the spine.

- The rocking motion challenges the coordination and balance of the body, enhancing overall body control.

- Hollow body rocking is commonly used in gymnastics and calisthenics training to develop a strong and stable core.

GOOD MORNING

- The good morning is a compound exercise that primarily targets the muscles of the lower back, hamstrings, and glutes.

- Proper form is crucial for good mornings to effectively engage the targeted muscles and prevent strain on the lower back. The movement involves hinging at the hips while keeping the back straight.

- Good mornings also engage the muscles of the core, including the erector spinae, obliques, and rectus abdominis.

- This exercise helps improve hip flexibility and mobility by emphasizing the hip hinge movement pattern.

- Good mornings can be performed with various tools, such as a barbell, dumbbells, or a resistance band, allowing for versatility in training.

- Including good mornings in a workout routine can contribute to increased posterior chain strength, including the muscles along the backside of the body.

- The exercise is effective for targeting the muscles responsible for maintaining an upright posture, promoting better spinal alignment.

- Good mornings can be adapted for different fitness levels by adjusting the load or the range of motion.

- The movement pattern in good mornings mimics certain aspects of daily activities, making it a functional exercise.

- Properly executed good mornings contribute to improved muscle imbalances in the lower back and hamstrings.

- The exercise can be used as a warm-up for the lower body or as part of a more comprehensive strength training program.

- Good mornings are considered a hip-dominant exercise, complementing knee-dominant exercises like squats.

JUMPING JACK

- Jumping jacks are a dynamic, full-body exercise that involves jumping to a position with the legs spread wide and the arms raised overhead, then returning to a position with the feet together and the arms at the sides.

- Jumping jacks are an excellent cardiovascular exercise that gets the heart rate up quickly, making them suitable for warm-ups, high-intensity interval training (HIIT), or as part of a cardio workout.

- This exercise engages multiple muscle groups, including the legs, core, arms, and shoulders.

- Jumping jacks are a low-impact exercise, making them accessible for individuals with joint concerns or those looking for a joint-friendly cardio option.

- Including jumping jacks in a workout routine can contribute to improved coordination and agility.

- Jumping jacks are versatile and can be modified to suit different fitness levels. Beginners can start with a slower pace or lower impact variations.

- The exercise promotes lymphatic drainage and can help with the circulation of oxygenated blood throughout the body.

- Jumping jacks can be part of a dynamic warm-up routine to increase body temperature and prepare the muscles for more intense physical activity.

- This exercise is often used in military training, group fitness classes, and as a component of calisthenics workouts.

- Jumping jacks can be incorporated into circuit training for a quick burst of cardiovascular activity between strength exercises.

- The rhythmic nature of jumping jacks can enhance mood and energy levels, making them a great addition to a workout for mental well-being.

DEADLIFT

- The deadlift is a compound exercise that targets multiple muscle groups, including the hamstrings, glutes, lower back, upper back, and forearms.

- Proper deadlift form involves lifting a barbell or other weighted object from the ground to a standing position, maintaining a straight back throughout the movement.

- Deadlifts are a functional exercise that mimics the lifting motion used in everyday activities, making them valuable for overall strength and mobility.

- Deadlifts are classified into various types, including conventional deadlifts, sumo deadlifts, Romanian deadlifts, and trap bar deadlifts, each emphasizing slightly different muscle groups and mechanics.

- The deadlift engages the posterior chain, which includes the muscles along the backside of the body, contributing to improved posture and spinal alignment.

- Deadlifts can be performed with various equipment, such as barbells, dumbbells, or kettlebells, providing versatility in training.

- This exercise is excellent for developing hip hinge mechanics, promoting better hip flexibility and mobility.

- Deadlifts are a compound movement that requires coordination and strength from various muscle groups, making them effective for building overall body strength.

- Including deadlifts in a workout routine can contribute to increased bone density, particularly in the spine and hip regions.

- Deadlifts are considered a powerlifting exercise and are often included in strength training programs to build maximum strength.

- The exercise also engages the grip and forearm muscles, contributing to improved grip strength.

T-BAR ROW

- T-bar rows are a compound exercise that primarily targets the muscles of the upper back, including the latissimus dorsi, rhomboids, and traps.

- The T-bar row is typically performed using a T-bar row machine, where a barbell is anchored at one end and weight plates are added to the other end.

- Proper form is crucial for T-bar rows to effectively engage the targeted muscles and prevent strain on the lower back. The back should be kept straight, and the movement should be initiated by pulling the elbows back.

- T-bar rows allow for a greater range of motion compared to some other rowing exercises, promoting better muscle activation.

- This exercise also engages the biceps, rear deltoids, and various muscles of the forearm.

- The T-bar row machine can be adjusted to accommodate different body sizes and preferences, allowing for a customized workout experience.

- T-bar rows are suitable for individuals looking to build upper back strength and muscle mass.

- Gripping the handles with a pronated (overhand) or neutral grip can target different areas of the upper back and biceps.

- T-bar rows can be included in both hypertrophy-focused and strength-focused training programs.

- Performing T-bar rows with proper technique contributes to improved posture by strengthening the muscles responsible for scapular retraction.

- Adding variations such as pause reps or adjusting the grip width can add complexity and intensity to T-bar row workouts.

- T-bar rows can be part of a well-rounded upper body workout routine, complementing pushing exercises like bench presses.

LAT PULLDOWN

- Lat pulldowns are a compound exercise that primarily targets the latissimus dorsi, the large muscles of the upper back.

- The exercise is typically performed on a cable machine with a high pulley, and the person pulls the bar down towards the upper chest.

- Proper form is crucial for lat pulldowns to effectively engage the targeted muscles. The back should be kept straight, and the movement should be initiated by pulling the elbows down and back.

- Lat pulldowns also engage the muscles in the arms, including the biceps, as well as the muscles in the shoulders.

- This exercise allows for a variety of grip positions, including wide grip, medium grip, and reverse grip, providing versatility in targeting different areas of the back and arms.

- Lat pulldowns are an effective alternative for individuals who may struggle with pull-ups, as they allow for controlled resistance and can be adjusted to different fitness levels.

- Including lat pulldowns in a workout routine can contribute to increased upper back strength and muscle development.

- The exercise promotes scapular retraction and protraction, enhancing overall shoulder stability and mobility.

- Lat pulldowns can be used as a warm-up exercise for the upper body, preparing the muscles for more intense activities.

- Adjusting the weight and rep range can make lat pulldowns suitable for both muscle hypertrophy and strength-building goals.

- Using various attachments, such as a straight bar or a V-bar, can provide different grip options and target the muscles from different angles.

- Lat pulldowns can be part of a comprehensive back workout routine, complementing other exercises like rows and deadlifts.

TRAP BAR WALK

- Trap bar walks, also known as trap bar farmer's walks, are a functional and full-body exercise that involves walking while carrying a trap bar loaded with weight.

- The trap bar is a hexagonal-shaped barbell that allows the individual to stand in the middle, providing a unique and comfortable grip for this exercise.

- Trap bar walks primarily target the muscles of the upper back, including the trapezius muscles, as well as the muscles in the shoulders, forearms, and core.

- Proper form is essential for trap bar walks to maximize muscle engagement and prevent unnecessary strain on the lower back. The individual should walk with a straight back and engage the core throughout the movement.

- Trap bar walks are an effective way to build grip strength, as the exercise requires holding onto the weighted bar for an extended period while walking.

- This exercise promotes stability and balance, as the individual must control the weight while moving.

- Trap bar walks can be adapted for different fitness levels by adjusting the weight or incorporating variations, such as walking on an uneven surface.

- Including trap bar walks in a workout routine contributes to improved posture by strengthening the muscles responsible for maintaining an upright position.

- The exercise can be part of a comprehensive strength training program, targeting the muscles of the upper back and core.

- Trap bar walks are a versatile exercise that can be performed as a standalone exercise or included in a circuit for a full-body workout.

BARBELL CURL

- Barbell curls are a classic isolation exercise that targets the biceps brachii, which is the muscle on the front of the upper arm.

- The exercise is performed by holding a barbell with an underhand grip and curling it toward the shoulders while keeping the upper arms stationary.

- Barbell curls engage not only the biceps but also the brachialis and brachioradialis muscles, contributing to overall arm development.

- Proper form is essential for barbell curls to effectively target the biceps and prevent unnecessary strain on the wrists and lower back. The movement should be controlled and deliberate.

- The exercise allows for variations in grip width, including a shoulder-width grip or a narrower grip, targeting the biceps from different angles.

- Barbell curls can be performed using an EZ-curl bar, which has a curved design to reduce strain on the wrists, or a straight barbell.

- Including barbell curls in a workout routine can contribute to increased bicep strength and muscle hypertrophy.

- This exercise is suitable for individuals at various fitness levels, and the weight can be adjusted based on individual strength and goals.

- Barbell curls are often used in bodybuilding and strength training programs to develop aesthetic arm muscles.

- The movement of barbell curls is a fundamental pattern for bicep training, and it can be used as a benchmark exercise to track progress.

- Performing barbell curls with proper technique helps to promote overall arm stability and control.

- Barbell curls can be included in superset or drop-set training techniques to add intensity to a workout.

SHRUG

- Shrugs are an isolation exercise that primarily targets the trapezius muscles, which run along the upper part of the back and neck.

- The exercise involves lifting the shoulders toward the ears, contracting the trapezius muscles.

- Proper form for shrugs includes maintaining a straight back and avoiding excessive neck movement to prevent unnecessary strain.

- Shrugs can be performed using various equipment, including dumbbells, barbells, or a Smith machine.

- The exercise can be executed with different grips, such as a pronated (palms facing the body) or neutral grip, to target the trapezius muscles from different angles.

- Shrugs are often incorporated into shoulder or upper body workouts to enhance overall muscle development.

- Including shrugs in a workout routine contributes to improved posture by strengthening the muscles responsible for scapular elevation.

- This exercise can be beneficial for individuals looking to develop a more defined and sculpted upper back.

- Shrugs are typically performed with relatively heavy weights, as the trapezius muscles respond well to resistance.

- The movement pattern in shrugs involves lifting the shoulders vertically, making it a straightforward and effective exercise.

- Shrugs are commonly used in bodybuilding and strength training programs to target the upper trapezius fibres.

- Beginners should start with a manageable weight and focus on controlled movements to avoid excessive strain on the neck and spine. Seeking guidance from a fitness professional can help ensure correct technique.

LATERAL RAISE

- Dumbbell lateral raises are an isolation exercise that targets the lateral or side head of the deltoid muscles, contributing to broader and more defined shoulders.

- The exercise involves lifting dumbbells laterally away from the body until the arms are parallel to the ground, creating a T-shape with the body.

- Proper form is crucial for dumbbell lateral raises to effectively engage the lateral deltoids and prevent unnecessary strain on the shoulders. The movement should be controlled, and the elbows should be slightly bent.

- Dumbbell lateral raises can be performed while standing or seated, providing versatility in training.

- Including lateral raises in a workout routine helps improve shoulder aesthetics by developing the side delts, contributing to a balanced shoulder appearance.

- The exercise engages the stabilizing muscles of the shoulders and upper back, promoting overall shoulder stability.

- Dumbbell lateral raises are suitable for individuals at various fitness levels, and the weight can be adjusted based on individual strength and goals.

- The lateral raise movement pattern can be adapted for variations, such as front raises or angled raises, to target the shoulders from different angles.

- Performing lateral raises with proper technique promotes better shoulder mobility and flexibility.

- Dumbbell lateral raises are often used in bodybuilding and aesthetic-focused training programs to enhance shoulder width.

- The exercise allows for a focused contraction of the lateral deltoids, making it effective for muscle hypertrophy.

SHOULDER PRESS

- The shoulder press, also known as the overhead press, is a compound exercise that primarily targets the deltoid muscles in the shoulders.

- The exercise involves lifting a weight, typically a barbell or dumbbells, from shoulder height to an overhead position.

- Proper form is crucial for shoulder presses to effectively engage the shoulders and prevent unnecessary strain on the neck and lower back. The movement should be controlled, and the core should be engaged for stability.

- Shoulder presses can be performed while standing or seated, offering variations in training.

- The exercise also engages the trapezius muscles, triceps, and various stabilizing muscles of the upper back.

- Including shoulder presses in a workout routine contributes to increased shoulder strength, promoting better functional strength for overhead activities.

- The shoulder press is a fundamental movement pattern for upper body strength and is often incorporated into strength training programs.

- Different grip widths and hand positions can be used in shoulder presses to target the shoulders from various angles.

- Seated shoulder presses with a backrest provide additional stability and support, reducing the strain on the lower back.

- The exercise can be performed with various equipment, including barbells, dumbbells, kettlebells, or even resistance bands.

- Shoulder presses are effective for developing muscle hypertrophy in the shoulders, contributing to a well-rounded and balanced physique.

- Including shoulder presses in a workout routine can help improve shoulder mobility and flexibility.

REAR DELT RAISE

- Rear delt raises are an isolation exercise that specifically targets the posterior or rear head of the deltoid muscles, which are located at the back of the shoulders.

- The exercise involves lifting dumbbells or other resistance away from the body in a horizontal plane, with the arms straight or slightly bent.

- Proper form is crucial for rear delt raises to effectively engage the posterior deltoids and prevent unnecessary strain on the shoulders. The movement should be controlled, and the shoulders should be kept down and back.

- Rear delt raises can be performed while lying facedown on an incline bench, seated, or bent over with the upper body parallel to the ground, providing versatility in training.

- Including rear delt raises in a workout routine helps to balance shoulder development, ensuring all heads of the deltoid muscles are targeted.

- The exercise engages the posterior deltoids, which play a crucial role in shoulder stability and overall shoulder health.

- Rear delt raises are suitable for individuals at various fitness levels, and the weight can be adjusted based on individual strength and goals.

- The movement pattern in rear delt raises can be adapted for variations, such as reverse flyes, to target the posterior deltoids from different angles.

- Rear delt raises are often used in bodybuilding and aesthetic-focused training programs to enhance the overall shape and definition of the shoulders.

- The exercise allows for a focused contraction of the rear deltoids, making it effective for muscle hypertrophy.

- Rear delt raises can be included in superset or drop-set training techniques to add intensity to a shoulder workout.

BENCH PRESS

- The bench press is a compound exercise that targets the chest, shoulders, and triceps muscles.

- The exercise is typically performed lying on a flat bench, lifting a barbell or dumbbells from chest level to a fully extended arm position.

- Proper form is crucial for bench presses to effectively engage the targeted muscles and prevent unnecessary strain on the shoulders and wrists. The back should be pressed into the bench, and the movement should be controlled.

- Bench presses can be performed with different grip widths, such as a wide grip or a narrow grip, to target the chest muscles from different angles.

- The exercise engages the pectoralis major, which is the large chest muscle, contributing to increased chest strength and muscle development.

- Including bench presses in a workout routine can help improve upper body strength and overall functional strength.

- The bench press is a fundamental movement pattern for upper body strength and is often incorporated into strength training and powerlifting programs.

- Variations of the bench press include the incline bench press (targeting the upper chest) and the decline bench press (targeting the lower chest).

- The exercise can be performed with various equipment, including barbells, dumbbells, or even resistance bands.

- Bench presses are effective for developing muscle hypertrophy in the chest, contributing to a well-rounded and balanced physique.

- Proper breathing technique, such as exhaling during the lifting phase and inhaling during the lowering phase, is important for optimal performance in bench presses.

CABLE CROSS OVER

- Cable crossovers are a cable machine exercise that targets the chest muscles, particularly the pectoralis major.

- The exercise involves standing in the centre of two cable machines with adjustable arms, pulling the handles or attachments across the body in a crisscross motion.

- Proper form is crucial for cable crossovers to effectively engage the chest muscles and prevent unnecessary strain on the shoulders. The movement should be controlled and deliberate.

- Cable crossovers provide constant tension on the chest muscles throughout the entire range of motion, making them effective for muscle activation and hypertrophy.

- The exercise allows for variations in hand position and angle, such as high, middle, or low cable positions, to target different areas of the chest.

- Cable crossovers are versatile and can be performed with different attachments, including single-hand grips, rope attachments, or wide bars.

- Including cable crossovers in a workout routine contributes to improved chest definition and aesthetics.

- The exercise engages the stabilizing muscles of the shoulders, promoting overall shoulder stability.

- Cable crossovers can be used as a finishing exercise in a chest workout, helping to enhance muscle pump and fatigue the chest muscles.

- Adjusting the cable height and angle allows individuals to emphasize either the upper, middle, or lower portion of the chest.

- Cable crossovers are suitable for individuals at various fitness levels, and the weight can be adjusted based on individual strength and goals.

INCLINE FLYE

- Incline flyes are a chest isolation exercise that targets the upper part of the pectoralis major muscles.

- The exercise is typically performed on an incline bench, with the individual lying face-up and holding dumbbells.

- Proper form is essential for incline flyes to effectively engage the upper chest muscles and prevent unnecessary strain on the shoulders. The movement should be controlled and deliberate.

- Incline flyes provide an effective stretch on the chest muscles at the bottom of the movement, contributing to muscle activation and hypertrophy.

- The exercise allows for variations in incline angles, such as low incline or high incline, to target different areas of the upper chest.

- Incline flyes are particularly beneficial for individuals looking to enhance the definition and development of the upper chest.

- The exercise engages the stabilizing muscles of the shoulders, promoting overall shoulder stability.

- Incline flyes can be performed with different hand positions, such as neutral grip or pronated grip, to target the chest from various angles.

- Including incline flyes in a workout routine helps to balance chest development and contributes to an overall aesthetically pleasing chest shape.

- The exercise can be part of a comprehensive chest workout, complementing other exercises like bench presses and cable crossovers.

- Incline flyes are suitable for individuals at various fitness levels, and the weight can be adjusted based on individual strength and goals.

- Incline flyes provide an alternative to flat bench flyes, emphasizing a different portion of the chest.

SQUAT

- Squats are a compound exercise that targets multiple muscle groups, including the quadriceps, hamstrings, glutes, and lower back.

- The squat is a fundamental movement pattern and a key exercise for building lower body strength and muscle mass.

- Proper form is crucial for squats to effectively engage the targeted muscles and prevent unnecessary strain on the knees and lower back. The movement involves bending at the hips and knees while maintaining a neutral spine.

- Squats can be performed with various equipment, including barbells, dumbbells, kettlebells, or bodyweight, providing versatility in training.

- Different squat variations include back squats, front squats, goblet squats, and overhead squats, each emphasizing slightly different muscle groups.

- Squats engage the core muscles as stabilizers, contributing to overall core strength and stability.

- Including squats in a workout routine can contribute to increased bone density, particularly in the hips and spine.

- The exercise promotes mobility and flexibility in the hips, knees, and ankles, enhancing overall lower body flexibility.

- Squats are known for their ability to elicit a strong hormonal response, promoting the release of growth hormone and testosterone, which are important for muscle growth and recovery.

- The movement pattern in squats mimics everyday activities like sitting and standing, making them functional for daily life.

- Squats can be adapted for different fitness levels by adjusting the depth of the squat and the resistance used.

- Including squats in a workout routine can contribute to improved athletic performance, as they are a key movement in many sports.

LEG CURL

- Leg curls are an isolation exercise that primarily targets the muscles of the hamstrings, which are located on the back of the thighs.

- The exercise involves flexing the knee joint to lift a resistance against the lower leg, typically using a leg curl machine.

- Proper form is crucial for leg curls to effectively engage the hamstrings and prevent unnecessary strain on the knee joints. The movement should be controlled, and the hips should be stabilized on the machine.

- Leg curls can be performed using various equipment, including seated or lying leg curl machines, resistance bands, or stability balls.

- Different leg curl variations include seated leg curls, lying leg curls, and standing leg curls, each targeting the hamstrings from slightly different angles.

- The exercise engages the muscles of the hamstrings, including the biceps femoris, semitendinosus, and semimembranosus.

- Including leg curls in a workout routine can contribute to balanced lower body development by targeting the often-neglected hamstrings.

- Leg curls are often used in rehabilitation programs for individuals recovering from hamstring injuries, as they provide controlled resistance to the muscles.

- The exercise promotes knee joint stability and flexibility by targeting the muscles responsible for knee flexion.

- Leg curls can be part of a comprehensive leg workout routine, complementing other exercises like squats and lunges.

- Proper breathing technique, such as exhaling during the lifting phase and inhaling during the lowering phase, is important for optimal performance in leg curls.

- Leg curls can be adapted for different fitness levels by adjusting the resistance, and they are suitable for both beginners and advanced athletes.

LEG EXTENSION

- Leg extensions are an isolation exercise that primarily targets the quadriceps muscles, located on the front of the thighs.

- The exercise involves extending the knee joint against resistance, typically using a leg extension machine.

- Proper form is crucial for leg extensions to effectively engage the quadriceps and prevent unnecessary strain on the knee joints. The movement should be controlled, and the back should be stabilized against the machine.

- Different leg extension variations include single-leg extensions, emphasizing one leg at a time, and standing leg extensions, providing additional stability challenges.

- The exercise engages the muscles of the quadriceps, including the rectus femoris, vastus lateralis, vastus medialis, and vastus intermedius.

- Including leg extensions in a workout routine can contribute to balanced lower body development by targeting the often-dominant quadriceps.

- Leg extensions are often used in rehabilitation programs for individuals recovering from knee injuries, as they provide controlled resistance to the quadriceps muscles.

- The exercise promotes knee joint stability and flexibility by targeting the muscles responsible for knee extension.

- Leg extensions can be part of a comprehensive leg workout routine, complementing other exercises like squats and lunges.

- Proper breathing technique, such as exhaling during the lifting phase and inhaling during the lowering phase, is important for optimal performance in leg extensions.

- Leg extensions can be adapted for different fitness levels by adjusting the resistance, and they are suitable for both beginners and advanced athletes.

CALF RAISE

- Calf raises are an isolation exercise that targets the muscles of the calves, specifically the gastrocnemius and soleus muscles.

- The exercise involves lifting the heels by pushing through the balls of the feet, emphasizing the contraction of the calf muscles.

- Proper form is crucial for calf raises to effectively engage the calves and prevent unnecessary strain on the ankles. The movement should be controlled, and the knees should be kept slightly bent.

- Calf raises can be performed using various equipment, including a calf raise machine, Smith machine, or a simple raised surface like a step or block.

- Different calf raise variations include standing calf raises, seated calf raises, and donkey calf raises, each targeting the calves from slightly different angles.

- The exercise engages the gastrocnemius, which is the larger and more visible muscle of the calf, as well as the soleus, which is located underneath the gastrocnemius.

- Including calf raises in a workout routine can contribute to improved calf development, enhancing the overall aesthetics of the lower leg.

- Calf raises are often used in sports-specific training programs, as strong and well-developed calves are essential for activities such as running and jumping.

- The exercise promotes ankle stability and flexibility by targeting the muscles responsible for plantarflexion.

- Calf raises can be part of a comprehensive lower body workout routine, complementing other exercises like squats and lunges.

- Proper breathing technique, such as exhaling during the lifting phase and inhaling during the lowering phase, is important for optimal performance in calf raises.

BARBELL AB ROLLOUT

- Barbell ab rollouts are a challenging core exercise that targets the muscles of the abdominal region, particularly the rectus abdominis.

- The exercise involves using a barbell with weight plates on the ends and rolling it away from the body while maintaining a plank position.

- Proper form is crucial for barbell ab rollouts to effectively engage the core and prevent unnecessary strain on the lower back. The movement should be controlled, and the core should be tight throughout.

- Barbell ab rollouts can be performed with various barbell types, including straight bars and curl bars, offering different grip options.

- The exercise engages not only the rectus abdominis but also the deep stabilizing muscles of the core, including the transverse abdominis.

- Including barbell ab rollouts in a workout routine can contribute to improved core strength, stability, and muscle endurance.

- Barbell ab rollouts are an effective progression from traditional ab rollouts using an ab wheel, adding additional resistance to the exercise.

- The movement pattern in barbell ab rollouts mimics the anti-extension function of the core, which is essential for maintaining spinal stability.

- Barbell ab rollouts are often used in strength and conditioning programs for athletes seeking enhanced core strength and functionality.

- The exercise can be adapted for different fitness levels by adjusting the weight on the barbell and the starting position of the rollout.

- Proper breathing technique, such as exhaling during the rolling out phase and inhaling during the return phase, is important for optimal performance in barbell ab rollouts.

- Barbell ab rollouts can be part of a comprehensive core workout routine, complementing other exercises like planks, Russian twists, and leg raises.

CABLE WOOD CHOP

- Cable wood chops are a functional and dynamic exercise that engages multiple muscle groups, including the core, obliques, shoulders, and hip muscles.

- The exercise involves using a cable machine with an adjustable pulley to mimic the chopping motion, starting high and moving diagonally downward.

- Proper form is essential for cable wood chops to effectively engage the targeted muscles and prevent unnecessary strain on the back. The movement should be controlled, and the core should be engaged throughout.

- Cable wood chops can be performed in various directions, including high-to-low and low-to-high, providing versatility in training.

- The exercise promotes rotational strength and stability, which is important for various sports and daily activities that involve twisting movements.

- Cable wood chops are suitable for individuals of different fitness levels, and the weight can be adjusted based on individual strength and goals.

- Including cable wood chops in a workout routine can contribute to improved functional fitness and overall core strength.

- The exercise engages the obliques, which are the muscles on the sides of the torso, contributing to better waistline definition.

- Cable wood chops are effective for targeting the muscles of the entire core, including the rectus abdominis and the deep stabilizing muscles.

- Proper breathing technique, such as exhaling during the chopping phase and inhaling during the return phase, is important for optimal performance in cable wood chops.

- Cable wood chops can be part of a comprehensive core workout routine, complementing other exercises like planks, Russian twists, and leg raises.

DECLINE SIT-UP

- Decline sit-ups are an abdominal exercise that targets the rectus abdominis, the muscles on the front of the abdomen.

- The exercise involves lying on a decline bench with the upper body positioned lower than the legs, securing the feet under foot pads, and performing a sit-up motion.

- Proper form is crucial for decline sit-ups to effectively engage the abdominal muscles and prevent unnecessary strain on the lower back. The movement should be controlled, and the core should be engaged throughout.

- Decline sit-ups increase the range of motion compared to traditional sit-ups, providing a more challenging workout for the abdominal muscles.

- The exercise engages not only the rectus abdominis but also the hip flexors and the muscles of the lower abdomen.

- Decline sit-ups can be adapted for different fitness levels by adjusting the decline angle or adding resistance, such as holding a weight plate against the chest.

- Including decline sit-ups in a workout routine can contribute to improved abdominal strength and muscle definition.

- The exercise involves a dynamic movement pattern, making it suitable for individuals looking to add variety to their core training.

- Decline sit-ups can be part of a comprehensive abdominal workout routine, complementing other exercises like planks, leg raises, and oblique exercises.

- Proper breathing technique, such as exhaling during the lifting phase and inhaling during the lowering phase, is important for optimal performance in decline sit-ups.

- The decline position shifts the focus of the sit-up motion, emphasizing the upper portion of the rectus abdominis.

DONKEY KICK

- Donkey kicks are a bodyweight exercise that targets the glutes, hamstrings, and lower back.

- The exercise involves starting on hands and knees in a tabletop position, lifting one leg and extending it upward toward the ceiling in a kicking motion.

- Proper form is crucial for donkey kicks to effectively engage the targeted muscles and prevent unnecessary strain on the lower back. The movement should be controlled, and the core should be engaged throughout.

- Donkey kicks primarily target the gluteus maximus, the largest muscle in the buttocks, helping to strengthen and tone the rear.

- The exercise engages the hamstrings as the leg is lifted, contributing to improved muscle definition in the back of the thighs.

- Donkey kicks can be performed with variations, including straight leg kicks, bent knee kicks, or pulses, to provide different challenges to the glutes and hamstrings.

- Including donkey kicks in a workout routine can contribute to improved hip stability and mobility.

- The exercise promotes isometric contraction in the glutes, which is essential for activities like walking, running, and climbing stairs.

- Donkey kicks are suitable for individuals at various fitness levels, and the intensity can be adjusted based on individual strength and goals.

- Donkey kicks can be part of a comprehensive lower body workout routine, complementing other exercises like squats, lunges, and leg lifts.

- Proper breathing technique, such as exhaling during the lifting phase and inhaling during the lowering phase, is important for optimal performance in donkey kicks.

CRUNCH

- Crunches are a popular abdominal exercise that targets the rectus abdominis, the muscles on the front of the abdomen.

- The exercise involves lying on the back with knees bent and feet flat on the ground, lifting the upper body off the floor using the abdominal muscles.

- Proper form is crucial for crunches to effectively engage the abdominal muscles and prevent unnecessary strain on the neck and lower back. The movement should be controlled, and the chin should be kept off the chest.

- Crunches are often included in abdominal workouts to improve core strength and muscle definition.

- The exercise engages the upper portion of the rectus abdominis, providing a targeted contraction for the "six-pack" muscles.

- Different variations of crunches include reverse crunches, bicycle crunches, and oblique crunches, each targeting different areas of the abdominal region.

- Crunches are a bodyweight exercise, making them accessible for individuals of various fitness levels.

- Including crunches in a workout routine can contribute to improved posture by strengthening the core muscles.

- The exercise can be performed with different hand positions, such as placing the hands behind the head or crossing them over the chest.

- Crunches can be part of a comprehensive core workout routine, complementing other exercises like planks, leg raises, and twists.

- Proper breathing technique, such as exhaling during the lifting phase and inhaling during the lowering phase, is important for optimal performance in crunches.

BICYCLE CRUNCH

- Bicycle crunches are a dynamic abdominal exercise that targets the rectus abdominis, obliques, and hip flexors.

- The exercise involves lying on the back, lifting the legs off the ground, and bringing one knee toward the chest while simultaneously rotating the torso to bring the opposite elbow toward the lifted knee.

- Proper form is crucial for bicycle crunches to effectively engage the abdominal muscles and prevent unnecessary strain on the neck and lower back. The movement should be controlled, and the lower back should be pressed into the floor.

- Bicycle crunches are known for their effectiveness in activating multiple muscle groups in the abdominal region, providing a comprehensive core workout.

- The exercise engages both the upper and lower portions of the rectus abdominis, contributing to overall core strength and definition.

- Performing bicycle crunches at a controlled pace with a focus on proper form enhances the effectiveness of the exercise.

- Bicycle crunches are an excellent choice for individuals looking to add variety to their abdominal workout routine.

- The exercise promotes rotational movement, which is important for functional core strength and stability.

- Including bicycle crunches in a workout routine can contribute to improved coordination and balance.

- The exercise allows for variations in intensity by adjusting the speed and range of motion.

- Bicycle crunches can be part of a comprehensive core workout routine, complementing other exercises like planks, leg raises, and traditional crunches.

DEAD BUG

- Dead bug exercises are a core workout that targets the rectus abdominis, obliques, and hip flexors.

- The exercise involves lying on the back with arms extended toward the ceiling and legs lifted off the ground. The movement includes extending one arm backward while lowering the opposite leg toward the floor and then alternating sides.

- Proper form is crucial for dead bug exercises to effectively engage the core muscles and prevent unnecessary strain on the lower back. The lower back should remain pressed into the floor, and the movements should be controlled.

- Dead bug exercises are known for promoting core stability and coordination by challenging the body to maintain a neutral spine while moving the limbs.

- The exercise engages the deep stabilizing muscles of the core, including the transverse abdominis, which contributes to overall core strength.

- Dead bug variations can include straight-leg dead bugs, bent-knee dead bugs, or adding resistance with a stability ball or resistance bands.

- The exercise helps improve the mind-muscle connection by requiring conscious control of limb movements while stabilizing the core.

- Including dead bug exercises in a workout routine can contribute to better posture and spinal alignment.

- Dead bug exercises are suitable for individuals at various fitness levels, and the difficulty can be adjusted based on individual strength and goals.

- The exercise promotes both flexion and extension of the limbs, making it a dynamic and effective core workout.

- Dead bug exercises can be part of a comprehensive core workout routine, complementing other exercises like planks, leg raises, and twists.

WINDSHIELD WIPER

- Windshield wiper exercises are an advanced core workout that targets the obliques, rectus abdominis, and hip flexors.

- The exercise involves lying on the back with arms extended outward for stability, lifting the legs toward the ceiling, and moving the legs in a controlled side-to-side motion, resembling the movement of windshield wipers.

- Proper form is crucial for windshield wiper exercises to effectively engage the core muscles and prevent unnecessary strain on the lower back. The lower back should remain pressed into the floor, and the movements should be controlled.

- Windshield wiper exercises challenge both the strength and flexibility of the core, requiring coordination and control during the rotational movement.

- The exercise engages the obliques, which are the muscles on the sides of the torso, contributing to improved waistline definition.

- Windshield wiper variations can include straight-leg windshield wipers or bent-knee windshield wipers, allowing individuals to adjust the difficulty level based on their fitness level.

- The exercise promotes rotational strength, which is important for activities that involve twisting and turning.

- Including windshield wiper exercises in a workout routine can contribute to improved core stability and spinal mobility.

- Windshield wiper exercises are suitable for individuals who have a strong core foundation and are looking for a challenging variation to add to their routine.

- The exercise requires a strong mind-muscle connection to maintain control over the leg movements while stabilizing the core.

- Windshield wiper exercises can be part of a comprehensive core workout routine, complementing other exercises like planks, leg raises, and twists.

INVERTED CURL

- Inverted curls typically target the muscles of the upper body, including the biceps, forearms, and the muscles of the back.

- Inverted curls can be performed with minimal equipment, often requiring a stable horizontal bar or the top edge of a door frame.

- Position yourself underneath the horizontal bar or door frame. Grasp the bar with an underhand grip, and your body should be at a slight angle, leaning back.

- Perform a curling motion by pulling your chest up towards the bar, engaging the biceps and forearms. Lower yourself back down with control.

- Inverted curls can be modified by adjusting the grip width, changing hand positions, or altering body angles to target different muscle groups.

- This exercise is effective for developing strength and definition in the biceps and forearms. It also engages the muscles of the upper back.

- Inverted curls can be adapted to different fitness levels. Beginners may start with a higher bar, while more advanced individuals can lower the bar or elevate their feet for added resistance.

- Ensure that the horizontal bar or door frame is stable and can support your body weight. Perform the exercise with controlled movements to avoid strain on the wrists and maintain proper form.

- Inverted curls can be incorporated into a full-body workout routine or included as part of a bodyweight exercise circuit.

- The number of repetitions and sets can vary based on individual fitness goals. Beginners may start with higher reps and lower sets, gradually progressing to more challenging variations.

- Prioritize a proper warm-up, including dynamic stretches and wrist mobility exercises, to prepare the muscles for the demands of inverted curls.

TRICEPS EXTENSION

- Triceps extension exercises primarily target the triceps brachii muscles, which are located on the back of the upper arm.

- Triceps extensions can be performed using various equipment, including dumbbells, barbells, cables, or machines. Common variations include overhead triceps extensions, lying triceps extensions, and triceps kickbacks.

- Triceps extensions involve the extension of the elbow joint, with the triceps muscles contracting to straighten the arm.

- Triceps extensions are considered isolation exercises, focusing on the targeted muscles without significant involvement of other muscle groups.

- Proper form is crucial to prevent strain on the elbows and wrists. Controlled movements, especially during the lowering phase, help maximize muscle engagement.

- Overhead triceps extensions involve lifting a weight overhead and extending the elbows. This variation places a greater emphasis on the long head of the triceps.

- In lying triceps extensions, performed on a flat bench, the barbell or dumbbells are lowered toward the forehead before being extended back up. This variation emphasizes the medial and lateral heads of the triceps.

- Triceps kickbacks involve extending the arm backward while holding a weight, emphasizing the contraction of the triceps muscles.

- Cable machines allow for constant tension on the triceps throughout the range of motion, providing effective muscle activation.

- Both dumbbell and barbell triceps extensions offer unique advantages. Dumbbells allow for greater freedom of movement and can help address muscle imbalances, while barbells provide stability and allow for heavier loads.

CRAB WALK

- Crab walks primarily target the muscles of the lower body, including the quadriceps, hamstrings, glutes, and hip abductors.

- To perform crab walks, sit on the floor with your hands behind you, fingers pointing away from your body. Lift your hips off the ground, supporting your weight on your hands and feet.

- Move laterally by walking with your hands and feet, maintaining the elevated hip position. The crab walk involves both forward and backward movements.

- Crab walks can elevate the heart rate and provide cardiovascular benefits, making them a dynamic and engaging exercise.

- The exercise engages the core muscles, especially the rectus abdominis and obliques, to stabilize the body during movement.

- Crab walks require hip mobility, helping to improve flexibility and range of motion in the hip joint.

- Crab walks can be adapted to different fitness levels by adjusting the speed, range of motion, or incorporating resistance, such as ankle weights or resistance bands.

- Crab walks can be included in a warm-up routine to activate the lower body muscles and prepare the joints for more intense exercises.

- Performing crab walks challenges coordination and balance, as the movement requires synchronizing the actions of the hands and feet.

- Reverse crab walks involve moving backward instead of forward, providing a different challenge to the muscles and coordination.

- Crab walks can be part of a comprehensive lower body workout routine, serving as a bodyweight exercise or a dynamic warm-up.

- Proper foot placement is essential for stability during crab walks. Ensure that the weight is evenly distributed between the hands and feet.

INCHWORM

- Inchworm exercises engage multiple muscle groups, including the core, shoulders, chest, arms, hamstrings, and lower back.

- Begin in a standing position with feet hip-width apart and hinge at the hips, bending forward to touch the floor with your hands.

- Walk your hands forward until you are in a plank position, maintaining a straight line from head to heels. Then, walk your feet towards your hands, returning to the bent-over position.

- Inchworms provide a dynamic stretch for the hamstrings and lower back during the forward fold.

- The plank position in the middle of the movement engages the core muscles, promoting stability and strength.

- The walkout phase of inchworms helps build shoulder and arm strength, especially in the deltoids and triceps.

- Inchworms can be progressed by incorporating a push-up when in the plank position or adding a jump at the end to turn it into an inchworm with a jump.

- Regular practice of inchworms can contribute to improved flexibility in the hamstrings and overall mobility.

- Inchworms, when performed at a faster pace, can elevate the heart rate, providing cardiovascular benefits.

- Inchworms can be adapted to different fitness levels by adjusting the speed, incorporating variations, or adding resistance through dumbbells or resistance bands.

- Inchworms are an effective warm-up exercise, preparing the body for more intense physical activity by increasing blood flow and activating various muscle groups.

BEAR CRAWL

- Bear crawls engage multiple muscle groups, including the shoulders, arms, core, hips, and legs, making them an effective full-body exercise.

- Begin on your hands and knees, with wrists directly under shoulders and knees under hips.

- Lift your knees a few inches off the ground and crawl forward by moving the opposite hand and foot simultaneously.

- Bear crawls challenge coordination and balance as you maintain a stable position on all fours while moving.

- The dynamic nature of bear crawls elevates the heart rate, providing cardiovascular benefits and contributing to overall fitness.

- The core muscles are heavily engaged during bear crawls to stabilize the body and maintain proper form.

- Bear crawls build upper body strength, particularly in the shoulders, triceps, and chest.

- The legs are activated during bear crawls, especially the quadriceps and hip muscles.

- Bear crawls can be adapted for different fitness levels by adjusting the speed, increasing the distance travelled, or incorporating variations like lateral or backward bear crawls.

- Bear crawls encourage a neutral spine position, promoting back health and reducing the risk of injury.

- Bear crawls are a functional exercise that mimics crawling movements, making them beneficial for athletes in various sports.

- Incorporating bear crawls into a workout routine can enhance agility and coordination, translating to improved overall athletic performance.

PLANCHE

- The planche is an advanced bodyweight exercise that originated in gymnastics and requires significant strength, balance, and flexibility.

- Planche exercises primarily target the upper body, engaging the shoulders, chest, triceps, and core muscles.

- The planche involves holding the body in a horizontal position with the arms straight, parallel to the ground, and the feet off the ground.

- Planche exercises come in different progression levels, from tuck planche to advanced variations like straddle planche and full planche.

- Achieving and maintaining the planche position requires exceptional core strength to keep the body parallel to the ground.

- Wrist strength and flexibility are crucial for planche exercises, as the body is supported on the hands with extended wrists.

- The shoulders play a significant role in planche exercises, providing the stability necessary to hold the body in the horizontal position.

- Planche exercises require a high level of balance and coordination, as the body is held without support points underneath.

- Achieving advanced planche variations often involves a good degree of flexibility, especially in the shoulders, hip flexors, and lower back.

- Mastering the planche typically involves progressive training, starting with easier progressions and gradually advancing to more challenging variations.

- Planche exercises emphasize body control and mastery over bodyweight, requiring a strong mind-muscle connection.

- Due to the advanced nature of planche exercises, there is an increased risk of injury, particularly to the wrists, shoulders, and lower back. Proper form and progression are crucial to minimize this risk.

BACK LEVER

- The back lever is an advanced bodyweight exercise that challenges strength, flexibility, and body control.

- Back lever exercises primarily target the muscles of the upper body, including the back, shoulders, chest, and arms.

- The back lever involves holding the body horizontally with the torso facing the ground and the arms fully extended, parallel to the ground.

- Like other advanced bodyweight exercises, the back lever has different progression levels, ranging from tuck back lever to advanced straddle or full back lever.

- Achieving and maintaining the back lever position requires significant core engagement to keep the body straight and horizontal.

- The exercise places a considerable demand on shoulder strength, especially in the muscles responsible for scapular retraction and depression.

- Grip strength is essential for the back lever, as the hands are typically positioned on a bar or rings during the exercise.

- Achieving the back lever often requires good wrist flexibility, as the wrists are extended during the movement.

- Back lever exercises emphasize body awareness and control, as the individual must maintain balance and stability throughout the movement.

- The back lever involves an inverted position, challenging individuals to become comfortable with being upside down and supporting their body weight.

- Due to the advanced nature of the back lever, there is an increased risk of injury, particularly to the shoulders, wrists, and lower back. Proper form, progression, and adequate warm-up are crucial to minimize this risk.

HUMAN FLAG

- The human flag is an advanced bodyweight exercise that challenges strength, stability, and body control.

- Human flag exercises primarily target the muscles of the upper body, including the core, shoulders, chest, and arms.

- The human flag involves holding the body horizontally while gripping a vertical pole or structure with the arms and keeping the body straight and parallel to the ground.

- Achieving the human flag is a progressive process, with variations ranging from tucked or straddled flags to the full human flag.

- Maintaining the human flag position requires exceptional core engagement to keep the body straight and parallel to the ground.

- The exercise places a significant demand on shoulder and arm strength, as the arms are used to support and stabilize the body.

- Grip strength is crucial for the human flag, as the hands grip a vertical pole or bar to support the body weight.

- The human flag heavily engages the oblique muscles, which play a key role in stabilizing the torso during the exercise.

- Achieving and holding the human flag requires a high level of balance and stability, as the body is suspended horizontally.

- Achieving the human flag often involves a good degree of flexibility, especially in the shoulders, hips, and lower back.

- Due to the advanced nature of the human flag, there is an increased risk of injury, particularly to the shoulders, wrists, and lower back. Proper form, progression, and adequate warm-up are crucial to minimize this risk.

- Consistent training and progressive overload are essential for achieving and progressing in human flag exercises. Building the necessary strength and stability takes time.

JUMP SQUAT

- Jump squats are a dynamic lower body exercise that combines the traditional squat movement with an explosive jump.

- The exercise primarily targets the muscles of the lower body, including the quadriceps, hamstrings, glutes, and calves.

- Jump squats elevate the heart rate, providing cardiovascular benefits and contributing to overall fitness.

- The explosive jump in jump squats helps develop lower body power, improving the ability to generate force quickly.

- Jump squats are a type of plyometric exercise, incorporating quick and powerful movements to enhance muscular performance.

- The core muscles are engaged during jump squats to stabilize the body during the squat and jump phases.

- The dynamic nature of jump squats increases caloric expenditure, making them an effective exercise for those looking to burn calories and improve body composition.

- Weight-bearing exercises like jump squats contribute to improved bone density, promoting overall bone health.

- Jump squats can be adapted for different fitness levels by adjusting the depth of the squat, jump height, or incorporating variations such as tuck jumps or split squat jumps.

- Jump squats can be included in various workout routines, such as circuit training, HIIT (high-intensity interval training), or as part of a dynamic warm-up.

- Regular inclusion of jump squats in a training program can lead to improved explosive strength and athletic performance.

- Landing softly and with proper technique is crucial to minimize impact on the joints and reduce the risk of injury during jump squats.

TUCK JUMP

- Tuck jumps are a dynamic plyometric exercise that involves explosive jumping and pulling the knees toward the chest in mid-air.

- Tuck jumps primarily target the lower body muscles, including the quadriceps, hamstrings, glutes, and calves. The core muscles are also engaged during the tucking motion.

- Tuck jumps elevate the heart rate, providing cardiovascular benefits and contributing to improved endurance.

- The explosive nature of tuck jumps helps develop lower body power, improving the ability to generate force quickly.

- Tuck jumps are a type of plyometric training, focusing on quick, powerful movements to enhance muscular performance.

- Due to their intensity, tuck jumps increase caloric expenditure, making them effective for burning calories and supporting weight management.

- Regular practice of tuck jumps can contribute to improved vertical jump height, making them beneficial for athletes involved in sports like basketball or volleyball.

- Tuck jumps require coordination and balance, especially during the tucking phase. They help improve overall body awareness and control.

- Tuck jumps can be adapted for different fitness levels by adjusting the intensity, jump height, or incorporating variations like double tuck jumps or alternating leg tuck jumps.

- Tuck jumps can be included in various workout routines, such as high-intensity interval training (HIIT), circuit training, or as part of a dynamic warm-up.

- Regular inclusion of tuck jumps in a training program can lead to improved explosive strength, which is beneficial for activities requiring quick and powerful movements.

CLAPPING PUSH UP

- Clapping push-ups are a dynamic variation of traditional push-ups that involve an explosive upward movement with a clap in mid-air.

- Clapping push-ups primarily target the muscles of the chest, shoulders, and triceps, with additional engagement of the core and stabilizing muscles.

- Clapping push-ups are a plyometric exercise, incorporating quick, powerful movements to enhance muscular performance and explosive strength.

- The explosive nature of clapping push-ups elevates the heart rate, providing cardiovascular benefits and contributing to improved endurance.

- Clapping push-ups help develop explosive upper body power, enhancing the ability to generate force quickly.

- Due to their intensity, clapping push-ups increase caloric expenditure, making them effective for burning calories and supporting weight management.

- Clapping push-ups can be adapted for different fitness levels by adjusting the intensity, incorporating variations like double claps, or performing them from different hand positions.

- Clapping push-ups can be included in various workout routines, such as high-intensity interval training (HIIT), circuit training, or as part of an upper body strength workout.

- Regular practice of clapping push-ups can lead to improved upper body strength, particularly in the chest, shoulders, and triceps.

- Clapping push-ups require coordination and precise timing to execute the explosive clap in mid-air, enhancing overall body awareness.

- Performing clapping push-ups with proper form is crucial to prevent injury. Landing softly and with control is essential to reduce stress on the wrists and shoulders.

LATERAL JUMP

- Lateral jumps are dynamic exercises that involve jumping laterally (side to side), engaging multiple muscle groups in the lower body.

- Lateral jumps primarily target the muscles of the legs, including the quadriceps, hamstrings, glutes, and calves. The lateral movement also engages stabilizing muscles.

- Lateral jumps elevate the heart rate, providing cardiovascular benefits and contributing to improved endurance.

- The lateral nature of the movement helps develop explosive power in the lower body, enhancing lateral strength and agility.

- Lateral jumps are a type of plyometric exercise, incorporating quick and powerful movements to enhance muscular performance.

- Lateral jumps require coordination and balance, especially during the take-off and landing phases. Regular practice can improve overall body awareness.

- Due to their intensity, lateral jumps increase caloric expenditure, making them effective for burning calories and supporting weight management.

- Lateral jumps can be adapted for different fitness levels by adjusting the intensity, distance jumped, or incorporating variations like lateral box jumps or lateral skater jumps.

- Lateral jumps can be included in various workout routines, such as high-intensity interval training (HIIT), circuit training, or as part of a dynamic warm-up.

- Regular practice of lateral jumps can contribute to improved agility and lateral movement, which can be beneficial for sports that involve quick changes in direction.

- Lateral jumps involve lateral movement, which can be good for joint health by promoting mobility and stability in different planes of motion.